BE
IRIE

BE IRIE

A Caribbean Handbook to Develop Healthy Habits

DR. KELENNE V. TUITT, MS, DO

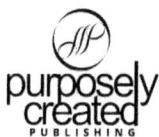

purposely
created
PUBLISHING

BE IRIE
Published by Purposely Created Publishing Group™
Copyright © 2019 Kelenne V. Tuitt

All rights reserved.

Printed in the United States of America
ISBN: 978-1-949134-90-2

Dr. Kelenne Tuitt's books and products are available through online book retailers.
To contact Dr. Kelenne Tuitt directly,
e-mail DrKelenne@mycaribbeandoctor.com

DEDICATION

To my mother, Lynett, who never let me settle for less, who guided me to greatness, and who has sacrificed to support me. I thank you and love you.

To my one and only son, Kaís. You are my world, and I push myself to make a better world for you and your future family to live in. You should want for nothing but understand that the true testament of a man is not what he has but what he gives.

To my Caribbean family. This book is for anyone born in the Caribbean, of Caribbean descent, or who just loves Caribbean food and culture. We as a people are full of life, energy, spontaneity, creativity, and love. We can make something beautiful from nothing. As a community, I want us to not only survive but to thrive. Being our best, challenging ourselves to reach higher levels, and never giving up are our strong points. However, to take on such a great task, we, my fellow bredredin and sistren, need to prioritize our health. Your health is your wealth. Success can only come from performing at your best, and to be your best, you should make time to take care of yourself. This book is here to show you that with simple lifestyle adjustments, you don't need to make time. Changing your mindset around food and exercise and consciously making healthier decisions while living your best life can be incorporated into your busy lifestyle. Thank you for taking time to read this book, as it's your first step to becoming the best you. In addition, you are supporting me on this journey of helping each Caribbean person achieve a healthier life. I am here to motivate you, guide you, and provide you a roadmap to success. As Trinidadians say, "Together we aspire. Together we achieve."

TABLE OF CONTENTS

Introduction 1

CHAPTER 1:
Top Diseases Affecting People of
Caribbean Descent 7

    1.1 Heart Disease 7

    1.2 Diabetes 9

    1.3 Cancer 11

    1.4 Stroke 12

CHAPTER 2:
Changing Our Mindset 19

    2.1 Visualization 20

    2.2 Realistic Expectations 22

    2.3 Bye Bye, Self-Sabotage 24

    2.4 Set Smaller Goals 26

    2.5 Ready, Set, Action! 29

2.6 Tracking Your Progress 31

2.7 Support 32

2.8 Rewards 34

CHAPTER 3:
It's Not a Diet, It's a Lifestyle 39

3.1 Food Groups 41

   3.1a Carbohydrates 41

   3.1b Vegetables 45

   3.1c Fruits 47

   3.1d Proteins 50

   3.1e Milk and Dairy Products 52

   3.1f Fats and Oils 54

3.2 Managing Cravings 55

3.3 Eating on the Go 57

3.4 Alcohol 58

CHAPTER 4:
Exercise 65

CHAPTER 5:
Preventative Health Screenings 75

   5.1 Well Adult Exam 76

       5.1a Male 77

       5.1b Female 78

   5.2 Mental Health 79

   5.3 Visual Health 80

   5.4 Foot Care 83

   5.5 Dental Care 83

   5.6 Hearing Protection 84

   5.7 Sexual Health 86

   5.8 Immunizations 88

   5.9 Dermatologic (Skin) Exam 88

CHAPTER 6:
Modern Medicine 95

BONUS 1:
Fitness Apps 101

BONUS 2:
Herbal Remedies 103

BONUS 3:
Health Benefits of Common Caribbean Drinks 107

Thank You 111

About the Author 113

INTRODUCTION

"Think like a queen. A queen is not afraid to fail. Failure is another stepping stone to greatness."

— **Oprah Winfrey**

Born on a small island in the Caribbean Sea called Trinidad, I was raised by my grandparents, mother, and extended family. I would run outside in the front yard to greet my neighbors and to see what was going on around the neighborhood. From what I was told, I would be ready to run off with my neighbors, as I was overly curious and adventurous. When I migrated to New York City, life was much different. No longer did coconut trees surround me with friendly neighbors who would greet me every morning; now I moved to an apartment in a cold concrete jungle. Despite the adjustment, my single mother made sure I felt comfortable. She made sure I was engaged and exposed to a multitude of opportunities. My mother encouraged me to go above and beyond. I was constantly told that education is your key to success because education affords you opportunity and access. I was very athletic and excelled in multiple sports while achieving top grades in a highly competitive International Baccalaureate program in high school. I was the president of the National Honor Society and had the distinguished honor of giving the high school graduation speech entitled "Soar Like An Eagle." In college, I worked three jobs while completing my Bachelor's in Biology with a pre-medical track. I also did a post-baccalaureate program in Biomedical Sciences and excelled to the top of my class. All of these experiences prepared me for that final goal I wanted to accomplish: becoming a doctor.

But why a doctor, you ask? During my summers, I would often travel to the Caribbean to visit my family, and it was heartbreaking to see my grandmother debilitated by a massive stroke. My grandfather and aunt cared for her the best way they could. My family even came together to bring her to America to seek advanced medical care, but it was too late. Being exposed to this had me curious about the human body and its ability to heal. I felt helpless in that situation, but that helplessness fueled my desire to learn, my desire to be the doctor who could help.

I used that fuel to excel in medical school until I got pregnant during my third year. I kept it to myself and pushed through. I did not want to answer the million questions such as, "What are you going to do? Are you taking time off?" Honestly, I didn't have any answers. All I knew was that this baby was inside of me and that he was safe. I really didn't want him to come out! Here I was with no job, homeless as I had to travel to different states for my clinical rotations, single, and pregnant. When I finally spoke with my school about my situation, they were accommodating and allowed me to complete rotations closer to home, where my mother assisted me with child care, and I graduated right on time. It was this blessing in the storm that pushed me to be the best physician I could be.

I would hold myself to a standard of treating each patient as family. I enjoyed listening to patients' stories about their grandchildren and providing a quiet moment of comfort as I held the hand of a recent widow. I loved celebrating my patients' wins, whether it was related to getting their sugar levels down or losing five pounds. I would go above and beyond to help a patient on a fixed income get the medications they need. That's what I would want my physician to do for my family or me.

As I started working for various organizations, I felt my values were compromised. I felt like a worker bee, just there to be productive. The focus was not on the quality of care; it was on the quantity. Patients are not objects, and they don't deserve to be treated like a task.

Patients deserved to be listened to, assessed properly, and have a thorough plan of care that is explained in a clear and concise manner that the patient understands and is motivated to participate in.

On the other hand, I was feeling overwhelmed and mentally exhausted. That's dangerous when caring for patients. Physicians need balance too. I was not finding time to exercise. I would eat fast food, as it was what was easily accessible and sometimes the only thing available. My health was deteriorating, and I was not my best self for my family or patients. So I made a decision to make a change. I took imperfect action and took back control of my life so that I could practice medicine on my terms while preserving my health.

So with this, I have chosen to create a life of flexibility, growth, and expansive reach on a global scale. I know the culture of Caribbean people, and many of them are skeptical of modern medication. They also tend to be busy people who make time for everyone else but themselves. I would like to help break those barriers and fuse both worlds of traditional and modern medicine. Education and access are the keys to doing this.

This book is designed to help Caribbean people and their decedents achieve optimal health on the go. No matter what your schedule may be, there is no excuse for you not to be at your optimal health. In order for you to be your best, your health must come first. It doesn't take a lot to maintain your health, but learning to prioritize your health will help you along the way.

I have too many friends with preventable diseases such as diabetes, high blood pressure, and high cholesterol. I have patients who have had heart attacks and strokes or who are on dialysis before the age of 40. Do you know someone who is on medication or should be? We all feel that we have tomorrow, but life is not guaranteed to any of us. We all have goals and aspirations. Peak performers have a routine and maintain their health. In order to do this, you need to have the right mindset and the right tools at your disposal. In this book, I am going to simplify and streamline the process.

CHAPTER 1

TOP DISEASES AFFECTING PEOPLE OF CARIBBEAN DESCENT

"If someone wishes for good health, one must first ask oneself if he is ready to do away with the reasons for his illness. Only then it is possible to help him."

—Hippocrates

1.1 HEART DISEASE

Cardiovascular (heart) disease is one of the leading causes of death globally. This group of diseases includes congestive heart failure (fluid build up), myocardial infarctions (heart attacks), irregular heart rhythms (i.e. atrial fibrillation or sick sinus syndrome where a pacemaker is needed), and valvular disease (leaky valves like mitral regurgitation or narrowed valves such as aortic stenosis). Oftentimes, patients are asymptomatic, or symptoms can be masked by other disorders. Symptoms include fatigue, weakness, dizziness, shortness of breath, chest pain, swelling of the lower extremities, the sensation that your heart is beating fast, or discomfort with exertion. Many times during a physical exam, a physician may be able to hear irregular heartbeats, however, most of the time, the heart rhythm and rate are normal.

There are several diagnostic tools we can use to identify the source of the problem. An electrocardiogram (EKG) may be used to see the electrical activity of the heart, namely how the heart beats. Another diagnostic tool is the echocardiogram. This is an ultrasound that is used to look at the structure of your heart and how well blood flows through the valves. If an abnormality is seen on either of the aforementioned tests, a more extensive evaluation called a cardiac stress test may be performed. This can be done manually by walking on a treadmill or chemically by using medication to speed up the rate of your heart. If there are abnormalities on your stress test, usually a cardiac catherization is done to look inside the blood vessels of the heart for blockages. Blockages occur when plaque builds up and prevents the circulation of blood to the heart. Just like any other muscle in our body, the heart needs oxygen. Without oxygen, the heart fatigues and the muscle cells die, leading to a heart attack.

1.2 DIABETES

"I always had to diet. I'm diabetic,
so it's a lifestyle for me anyway just to stay healthy
and not end up in the hospital."

—Halle Berry

Diabetes Mellitus comes in two forms: Diabetes Mellitus Type I and Diabetes Mellitus Type 2. Type 1 Diabetes Mellitus is considered to be an autoimmune disorder where your body attacks the pancreas, where insulin is produced and stored. Insulin helps to remove glucose (sugar) from your body. If the pancreas can no longer produce insulin, then your sugar goes up, and you can develop diabetes. Type 2 Diabetes Mellitus usually is a result of a poor diet and sedentary lifestyle. It can be prevented with the adoption of a healthy lifestyle. Type 2 Diabetes typically occurs later in life but can occur in children who have diets high in sugar. For purposes of this book, we will focus on Diabetes Type 2.

Diagnosing diabetes involves one of three tests. You can do a blood test called a HbgA1c. If a patient's HbgA1c is less than 5.7, they are considered to not be a diabetic. If your HgbA1c is between 5.8 and 6.4, you are considered borderline or pre-diabetic. An A1c greater than or equal to 6.5 is indicative of diabetes. The second test that can be done to diagnose diabetes is a fasting blood glucose test. After a patient fasts for eight or more hours, their blood is drawn. If your fasting blood glucose is over 126 mg/dL (7mmol/L) on two separate tests, you probably have diabetes. If you have a fasting blood glucose level of 100-125 mg/dL (5.6 – 6.9 mmol/L), you are considered pre-diabetic. The third test used to diagnose diabetes is an oral glucose tolerance test, where you fast overnight and your fasting sugar is measured. Then you drink a sugary drink, and your glucose levels are measured at specific intervals over a two-hour period. A blood glucose level less than 140 mg/dL (7.8 mmol/L) is normal. A reading above 200 mg/dL (11.1 mmol/L) is high and suggestive of diabetes. There are millions of patients who are unaware that they are pre-diabetic because they do not go for a general check up with a medical provider. Pre-diabetes is the most critical time where lifestyle adjustments can reverse the course of this illness.

There are many signs and symptoms of diabetes, and everyone has different experiences. Symptoms of diabetes include increased thirst, hunger, or urination. Having frequent and recurring infections such as urinary tract infections, yeast infections, or skin infections may prompt your physician to check you for diabetes. Having a cut that takes a long time to heal may also indicate diabetes. This is because diabetes damages the blood vessels and restricts blood flow, leading to delayed wound healing. You may also have numbness or tingling in your hands or feet, which is a sign of nerve damage. High blood sugar levels weaken nerve fibers, reducing sensation, which can also extend to major organs such as your heart, gastrointestinal system, and urinary system. Changes in your vision may be a sign of diabetes. Often when someone's blood sugar drops, they may have blurry vision. You can also develop cataracts, glaucoma, and even blindness from uncontrolled diabetes. You may feel fatigued easily or have mood swings due to fluctuations in your blood glucose level. Diabetics also have a higher risk of developing depression.

1.3 CANCER

In the Caribbean region, cancer is the second leading cause of mortality, with an estimated 87,430 cancer-related deaths reported in 2013.[1] Among males, prostate

---

1   Ref: Razzaghi H, Quesnel-Crooks S, Sherman R, et al. "Leading Causes of Cancer Mortality – Caribbean Region, 2003-2013." MMWR Morb Mortal Wkly Rep. 2016; 65(49):1395-1400

cancer was the leading cause of cancer deaths, followed by lung cancer, stomach cancer, and colorectal cancer. Among females, breast cancer was the most common cause of cancer deaths, followed by cervical cancer, lung cancer, and colorectal cancer. Lung cancer is the leading cause of cancer death in this region for both sexes combined.[2]

Lifestyle factors such as smoking tobacco products, excessive alcohol consumption, and unprotected sex also contribute to such conditions. Many of these conditions do not have symptoms until it is too late. Through education, awareness, screening initiatives, and proper follow-up, the incidence of such conditions can be reduced.

1.4 STROKE

Cerebral vascular accidents (strokes) occur when part of the brain loses oxygen. CVAs can affect people's speech and their ability to perform functions like walking and swallowing. There are ischemic strokes, where the arteries that carry oxygen to the brain are blocked. There are also hemorrhagic strokes, where a leaky or weak blood vessel in the brain ruptures. Some people can have a

---

2   Cancer in Latin America and Caribbean | Cancer Atlas

temporary disruption in blood flow to the brain where they have symptoms for less than 24 hours. There is no permanent damage. This is called a transient ischemic attack (TIA). There are many risk factors for strokes, including high blood pressure, high cholesterol, diabetes, sleep apnea, cigarette smoking, and family history of stroke or heart attack.

Being able to quickly identify the signs and symptom of a stroke can drastically improve the outcomes. Think "FAST":

a) **Face**: Ask person to smile. Does one side of the face droop?

b) **Arms**: Ask person to raise both arms. Does one arm drift downward or not move?

c) **Speech**: Ask the person to repeat a simple phrase like "The sky is blue." Is the person's speech slurred or strange?

d) **Time**: If you observe any of the symptoms above, call emergency services immediately.

Being able to identify these symptoms can be the difference between life and death. Other symptoms include:

a) Paralysis or numbness of the face, arm, or leg on one side of your body.

b) Trouble seeing out of one or both eyes.

c) Sudden onset of the worst headache of your life. You may have dizziness, nausea, or confusion associated with this.

d) Trouble walking.

If you notice any of these signs of symptoms or you are not sure, please go see your doctor. Some people may have slight symptoms for days. For others, symptoms come on suddenly. The sooner this is evaluated, the quicker intervention can be done to reduce the long-term effects of a stroke. Various imaging tools, such as an MRI or CT scan, are used to look at the brain and see the impact of the stroke. You may also have a cardiac evaluation or an ultrasound of your neck to identify the cause of the stroke.

The above are the top four diseases afflicting people of the Caribbean. Many are preventable through diet, exercise, and preventative screenings. Let's see how we can combat these processes together.

{ NOTES }

{ NOTES }

{ NOTES }

{ NOTES }

CHAPTER 2

CHANGING OUR MINDSET

*"Learning the mind is as important
as understanding the body."*

—**Usain Bolt**

Growing up in a Caribbean household means you eat all of your food on your plate. Nothing goes to waste. Many times, our grandparents may give us a "sweetie" after eating. At Christmas, we indulge in black cake (rum cake), sorrel, pastels, ham, lamb, chow—the list goes on. I'm getting hungry now just writing this list! There is nothing wrong with indulging once in a while, but when we get into the hustle and bustle of life, we tend to stray from our upbringing. The majority of modern-day Caribbeans do not have a stay-at-home mother who can cook three fresh meals a day and are instead navigating life the quick and easy way. With the Americanization of many of the islands and of course living in America, there is more access to a wide array of foods. We tend to get away from our roots and eat more processed food than natural foods on which we grew up. Before we can change our diet, we have to change our mindset around health. Here are some steps to get you started.

2.1 VISUALIZATION

Have you ever sat and daydreamed about what you want out of life? This is called visualization. You can actually feel how happy you are and see your success in having attained what it is you want. So why not use these skills to visualize your health? I want you to visualize your health over the next six to twelve months. Think about where you are now. Where do you want to be in six to twelve months? Visualize how you would feel. Visualize the comments your friends and family will give you. Visualize the confidence and swagger you will have. I want you to get old photos and use them as a reminder of where you want to be or don't want to be, depending on where you are on your journey. Get an old pair of jeans or buy a pair one size smaller. Once a month, try them on until you can fit them. Get in action. Write down your goals for next year.

Be Irie

2.2 REALISTIC EXPECTATIONS

Now that we have visualized our life of abundant health, let's get realistic about our expectations. Some of us want to be healthier, and many of us want to be skinner. Skinny does not equal healthy. I have many plus-size patients who are healthier than my petite patients. Aesthetically, a small waist and a six pack looks good, but how we get there is just as important. Quick diets and starvation do not solve the root issue. Neither does setting unrealistic expectations. This will set you up for failure. Your body does not rapidly gain weight over night (unless there is a medical issue). So losing weight over night will not happen either.

So what is a realistic goal for weigh loss? One to two pounds a week is attainable and will result in longer success. If you're new to this, you can say, "In one year, I want to be 12-24 pounds lighter." This is totally doable. This means losing one to two pounds a month or three to six pounds every quarter. It may not sound like much, but the results will impact your life drastically. You will feel lighter, your back and knees won't hurt as much, you will have more energy, and your confidence will increase as your clothing fits better.

Realistic expectations also include your actions. In my head, I may say, "Oh, I am waking up at 5 AM and running two miles every day for the next month." However, realistically, I'm not a morning person. And when is the last time I ran? This may be my ultimate goal, but to make it possible, I can say, "I plan to wake up and start walking for 20 minutes, three days a week, for the next month." This is doable; it helps to build my stamina so that when I do start running, I won't feel so defeated because of how out of shape I am. What do you think is reasonable for you to change to help you achieve your goals? Start by breaking it down into quarters. Write down your goals for each month of that quarter. At the end of each quarter, you can do an assessment.

2.3 BYE BYE, SELF-SABOTAGE

"Love the life you live. Live the life you love."

—**Bob Marley**

In order for you to achieve your realistic goals, you have to get rid of self-sabotage. These are the old habits that are contradictory to your desires. We know that these habits are not healthy, but we still do them. We come up with excuses for them. These are our guilty pleasures. Some of us just don't care and will do them because we feel like it. Some of us hide and do them in secret. When you engage in these habits, whether in secret or openly, you are not harming anyone but yourself. For example, I might go to the gym and work out for 30 minutes, then I come home and eat a bowl of ice cream. Another example would be eating a salad for lunch but then having a Snicker's bar. Or I know I'm not supposed to eat late at night, but I snack on cookies, chips, and soda before bed. Ask yourself why you might engage in these habits. If you desire sweets, then choose a lower calorie option, such as a handful of grapes or a sherbet. If it's because of boredom, then let's find something else to keep you busy. If it's because you just want it, then enjoy and forget what I'm saying because you're not ready to change your health. We all have habits that are hard to break, but if you really take the time to reflect about why you think you can't resist something, you can work on changing your mindset around it to make better decisions. I don't want you to deprive yourself, but making healthier decisions that give you that gratification you desire will help you achieve those goals you have set above. Identify five guilty pleasures you enjoy and write down how you're going to change them.

2.4 SET SMALLER GOALS

"You have to set yourself goals so you can push yourself harder. Desire is the key to success."

—Usain Bolt

Now, let's set some goals! We visualized and know what the end goal is. You never want to keep the big picture out of sight. You have identified your realistic expectations and will work on changing your old habits. However, to get there will be a process. Trust the process! Setting attainable goals each week will pay off. Each small win accumulates into huge success. Improving your lifestyle does not mean you have to interrupt your normal life. Here are some examples of simple steps that can fit into your normal life:

1. Take the stairs instead of the elevator.

2. Drink water instead of juice or soda.

3. Eat fruit instead of candy or cake.

4. Eat low-fat popcorn or vegetable chips instead of regular chips.

5. Have a salad with nuts, fruits, eggs, kale, and spinach. It's more nutritious and filled with proteins and vitamins.

6. Park your car farther from where you need to be.

7. Play some high-energy music and dance.

8. Don't sit at your computer for hours. Take a break every 45-60 minutes. Do 10 squats, 10 jumping jacks, and stretch.

9. Ride you bike.

10. Play outside. Do something fun like roller skating or rock climbing.

11. While watching TV, do some squats and arm curls with a can of peas in each hand.

12. When you wake up in the morning, stretch. Touch your toes, roll your waist, and do shoulder rolls.

What are some simple actions that can fit into your lifestyle?

Dr. Kelenne V. Tuitt, MS, DO

2.5 READY, SET, ACTION!

"Dreams are free. Goals have a cost. While you can daydream all day, goals don't come without a price: time, effort, sacrifice, and sweat!"

—Usain Bolt

Now you have a plan. Let's take action! Eighty percent of the battle is planning ahead. Be committed to this like you're committed to your job. You need money to survive, so you go to work. Well, you can't work unless you're healthy. Let's be clear: Your Health is Your Wealth! It doesn't make sense to work eight- to twelve-hour days for most days of the year, so that when you retire you can decide to finally live. By then, you may have high blood pressure, diabetes, arthritis, or other conditions that can hinder your health. We are going to live now! We are making a commitment to ourselves to be healthier, well rounded, and conscious about our decisions. We shouldn't only put thought into the things we do for other people. We need to be aware and thoughtful of what we do to and for ourselves.

We sat and visualized and planned, but now we have to take action. Action does not need to be an hour or more. Action can be the choices we make for lunch or dinner. Action can be exercising while watching our favorite TV show. Action can be incorporated into our daily activities. Action can involve our kids and family. Don't make excuses about your health. Think differently! We don't need to create the time. We have to maximize the time we have.

Forming new habits can take time. The old saying was that it takes 21 days to develop a new habit. However, that's not true. There are many variables that go into habit formation, but most important is your determination. Habits can take 18 to 254 days to form and become second nature. Regardless of where you are in your journey, as long as you don't give up, you're already winning. Let today be your first day of action!

Write two things you're going to do today. Check them off and post them on my Facebook fan page: www.facebook.com/drkelenne.

2.6 TRACKING YOUR PROGRESS

So now you have taken action. Let's see your progress. Before you start your journey, you should weigh yourself, take your measurements, and write down your Body Mass Index. You can get a sample tracker on my website www.DrKelenne.com. Take your measurements every quarter. Don't worry about the number on the scale. Muscle weighs more than fat. Some may tone up and lose inches, but their weight remains the same. Track how you feel. Do your clothes fit better? Can you now slide those old jeans that you want to fit into past your thighs? Hey, that's progress! We celebrate everything. Every success is a win.

There are several ways to track your progress. You can write it down in a journal or you can use an app. Check out the bonus section for a list of fitness apps that you can use.

2.7 SUPPORT

*"There is no greater agony than bearing an
untold story inside you."*

—Maya Angelou

Awesome! You have put your plans into action, but you can't lose momentum. Don't be shy! Share your journey. Let your friends, family, co-workers, and physician know. This is a form of accountability. The more people you have in your village supporting you, the more successful you become. They want to see you win just as much as you do. Write a blog about your journey. Some days will be hard, but a true measure of your success is how you overcame those trials. Don't keep your wins to yourself; share them. You never know who is watching and who you are inspiring. Share your wins with me on my Facebook page: www.facebook.com/DrKelenne.

Who is your support system? Don't keep your journey a secret! What will motivate you to overcome?

Be Irie

2.8 REWARDS

It's the end of the first month or the first quarter. You have reached your goal! You did it! Wow, that wasn't so bad. How are you going to celebrate? You deserve it. At the end of each month, treat yourself. Whether it is to a manicure, a new dress, movies, or shopping, do something. Try not to reward yourself with food, as we are trying to create a lifestyle of healthy choices, and emotional eating is not a part of that. List the rewards you want to attain:

{ NOTES }

{ NOTES }

{ NOTES }

{ NOTES }

CHAPTER 3

IT'S NOT A DIET, IT'S A LIFESTYLE

"A healthy lifestyle not only changes your body, it changes your mind, your attitude, and your mood."

—Anonymous

Let's get down to the basics. We learn how to eat from our parents. If your household was like mine, you finished what was given to you, as food is not meant to be wasted. However, does it matter what's on our plate or how much is on our plate? If it's a holiday, like Christmas, everyone's mouth is watering to taste the sweet aromas of all the special homemade treats in the air. This is when we tend to overindulge. Enjoying these moments once in a while is not a problem at all. In fact, I encourage it. However, the key words are *once in a while*. In order to enjoy these moments, we have to control our daily habits.

What we eat and how much we eat are both important. Most foods in the Caribbean are healthy, but it's how we prepare it that strips the nutrients. Some foods are full of calories, and when you overindulge, it can widen your waistline faster. You should eat for nourishment, not for fullness. It is not hard to maintain a healthy diet once you are aware of the foods that will help you and not harm you. We usually reach for what's familiar, but now we are going to change our mindset around food.

You are what you eat! No, you're not a pig if you eat pork. However, if you eat too much fried food, eventually, that cholesterol will build up in your arteries and lead to a heart attack or stroke. If you have to eat your rice and peas with jerk chicken and then wash it down with a soft drink daily, eventually that excess sugar will manifest into diabetes. Being aware of the types of foods there are, their portions, their calories, and their nutritious value will help you along the way. Let's learn about what we are eating and how they impact us.

3.1 FOOD GROUPS[3]

3.1a Carbohydrates

Carbohydrates such as breads, cereal, pasta, and rice are staples in our households. Carbohydrates are a major source of energy. However, not all carbohydrates are created equally. There are three types of carbohydrates: sugar, fiber, and starches. We can break them down further into simple and complex carbohydrates. Simple carbohydrates are broken down easily by the body. They can be found naturally in fruits or milks, or they can be refined and added to sodas, cakes, and candies. Complex carbohydrates are longer chains of sugar molecules that take longer to be broken down by the body, thus providing a more consistent stream of energy. They are found in whole grains, legumes (beans), and starchy vegetables. So which should you eat? Well, they are both good for you as long as you avoid processed sugars found in pastries, energy drinks, sodas, and ice cream. No, I'm not saying you can't ever eat these foods again. Eating these foods in moderation is okay, but on a daily basis, you

---

3   https://www.cnpp.usda.gov/sites/default/files/archived_projects/FGPPamphlet.pdf

want to eat more complex carbohydrates and simple sugars from fruits and vegetables.

Here are examples of simple carbohydrates you can integrate into your diet:

- Apples
- Cherries
- Honey
- Lemon
- Papaya
- Pineapple
- Plum
- Mango
- Strawberries
- Unsweetened 100 percent fruit juice

Here are examples of complex carbohydrates you want in your diet:

- Cabbage
- Spinach

- Cucumbers

- Oatmeal

- Brown Rice

- Whole Wheat Bread

- Wild Rice

- Quinoa

- Lentils

- Kidney Beans

- Chickpeas

- Carrots

- Okra

- Cassava

- Yam

Here are examples of simple carbohydrates you want to **avoid** in your diet:

- White Bread

- White or Brown Sugar

- White Rice

- Muffins

- Candy

- Cake

- Pretzels

- Chips

- Soda

- White Potatoes

A serving is usually one slice of bread, one ounce of cereal or half a cup of cooked rice or pasta. Having six to eleven servings of the right carbohydrates per day is reasonable.

Choosing carbohydrates with a high fiber content, such as 100 percent whole wheat bread, whole wheat pasta, or whole grain cereals, would be a better option. Brown rice can be used in place of white rice. When baking bread, use whole wheat flour. If purchasing bread, rice, or pasta, get a product with little fat or sugar.

3.1b Vegetables

Vegetables are a great source of vitamins and minerals that help us with our energy levels, vision, bone strength, skin clarity, digestive health, mental health, and cardiovascular health. They are naturally low in fat and high in fiber. It is recommended to have three to five servings a day. A serving can be one cup of raw leafy green vegetables like spinach, kale, broccoli, or cabbage or half a cup of cooked or raw vegetables like carrots, sweet potatoes, corn, or legumes (kidney beans or chickpeas). Some vegetables are starchy yet equally nutritious, such as eddo, yam, cassava, pumpkin, and boniato.

Here is a list of the most nutritious vegetables in the world:[4]

- Asparagus – High in folate, selenium, vitamin K, thiamin, and riboflavin

- Broccoli – Full of Vitamin K, C, folate, manganese, and potassium. It's also a sulfa-containing plant that has properties to protect against cancer

---

4   https://www.healthline.com/nutrition/14-healthiest-vegetables-on-earth

- Brussels Sprouts – High in Vitamins K, A, and C, folate, manganese, potassium, and antioxidants

- Carrots – Full of Vitamins A, K, and C, potassium, and antioxidants

- Collard Greens – Full of fiber, protein, and calcium. May also reduce the risk of glaucoma and prostate cancer

- Garlic – Can lower triglyceride levels and blood glucose levels and potentially protect against cancer

- Ginger – Helps with motion sickness, can help treat anti-inflammatory disorders such as lupus, gout, and arthritis, and potentially lower blood sugar levels

- Green Peas – High in protein, fiber, Vitamins A, C, and K, riboflavin, thiamine, niacin, and folate.

- Kale – High in Vitamins B, K, A, and C, copper, potassium, calcium, and antioxidants

- Red Cabbage – High in fiber, Vitamin C, and antioxidants. May reduce cholesterol levels

- Spinach – Full of Vitamins A and K and antioxidants

- Sweet Potato – High in fiber, protein, Vitamins C and B6, potassium, manganese, and beta-carotene, which can potentially reduce cancer. Ciapo (a specific type of sweet potato) may also reduce cholesterol and blood sugar levels.

- Swiss Chard – High in fiber, protein, Vitamins A, C, and K, manganese, magnesium, and antioxidants. Can help reduce effects of diabetes

3.1c Fruits

Fruits are a great substitute for that sweet tooth. They are full of water and are a great source of Vitamins A and C and potassium. They are low in fat and sodium. It is recommended to have two to four servings a day. A serving would be a medium apple, banana or orange; half a cup of chopped, cooked, or canned fruit; or three fourths of a cup of unsweetened 100 percent fruit juice. Try to select fresh fruits instead canned or frozen fruits in heavy syrups. Whole fruits have more fiber than fruit juices.

Here is a list of the world's healthiest fruits:[5]

❯ Grapefruit – Aids in weight loss, reduces insulin resistance.

❯ Pineapple – High in manganese. Also has anti-inflammatory properties that may reduce cancer risk.

❯ Avocado – High in magnesium, potassium, fiber, and healthy fats; low in carbohydrates. It also has cardiovascular benefits.

❯ Blueberries — High in fiber, Vitamins C and K, and manganese. Has the highest antioxidant content of all fruits.

❯ Apples – High in fiber, Vitamins C, K, and B-complex, potassium, and antioxidants. They also contain pectin, which is a fiber that feeds on the good bacteria in the gut and helps with digestive health.

❯ Pomegranate – Nutrient dense. High in antioxidants, which have anti-inflammatory properties and may reduce risk of cancer.

---

5   https://www.healthline.com/nutrition/20-healthiest-fruits#section1

❷ Mango – High in Vitamin C, soluble fibers, and antioxidants. Has anti-inflammatory properties.

❷ Strawberries – High in Vitamin C, manganese, folate, and potassium. They have a low glycemic index, meaning they don't spike your blood sugar levels.

❷ Cranberries – High in Vitamins C, E, and K1, copper, manganese, and antioxidants. Can help prevent urinary tract infections.

❷ Lemons – High in Vitamin C. It can potentially lower blood pressure and cholesterol levels, thus preventing cardiovascular disease.

❷ Durian (also known as the "king of fruits") — High in Vitamin C, manganese, B vitamins, copper, folate, manganese, and antioxidants.

❷ Watermelon – High in Vitamins A and C and antioxidants. It is also hydrating.

❷ Olives – High in Vitamin E, iron, copper, and calcium.

❷ Blackberries – High in Vitamin C, manganese, minerals, fiber, and antioxidants.

- Oranges – High in Vitamin C, potassium, B-complex, thiamine, and folate. They can also reduce the risk of kidney stones and help with iron absorption to prevent anemia.

- Bananas – High in potassium. The carbohydrates in green, unripe bananas are resistant starches, meaning that they function like fibers and are slower to digest. This can help with blood sugar control.

- Guava – High in Vitamins C and A, potassium, copper, manganese, fiber, folate, and antioxidants.

- Papaya – High in Vitamins C and A, potassium, folate, and antioxidants. Also helps with digestion.

- Cherries – High in potassium, fiber, Vitamin C, antioxidants, and melatonin, which helps you to sleep better.

3.1d Proteins

Proteins include meat, poultry, fish, eggs, dry beans, and nuts. They provide Vitamin B, iron, and zinc, which are all essential vitamins and minerals. It is recommended to have two to three servings a week. A serving is considered to be two to three ounces of cooked lean meat, poultry, or fish per day.

Examples of lean meats include:

> Beef – loin, sirloin, or round steaks/roast

> Pork Roasts/Chops – tenderloin, center loin ham

> Veal — all cuts except ground

> Lamb Roast/Chops — leg and loin

> Chicken and Turkey – light and dark meat without the skin

> Fish and Shellfish – Most are low in fat, however, those marinated or canned in oil have a higher fat content.

> Goat – Lower in calories, saturated fats, and cholesterol than beef, pork, lamb, and chicken.

> Oxtails – High in saturated fat. Eat sparingly.

These foods are also equivalent to one serving size of meat:

- ❯ Half a cup of beans – soybeans (edamame), lentils, split peas, pinto beans, kidney beans, black beans, lima beans.

- ❯ One egg — Avoid the yolk, as it is high in cholesterol. Egg whites have more protein.

- ❯ Two tablespoons of peanut butter

- ❯ A third of a cup of nuts/seeds – almonds, pumpkin seeds, sunflower seed, cashew nuts

3.1e Milk and Dairy Products

Dairy products provide protein, vitamins, and minerals, especially calcium, which is important for bone and cardiovascular health. It's recommended to have two to three servings a day. For pregnant women, breast-feeding mothers, and teenagers, three servings are recommended.

Here are some examples of healthy dairy products:

- ❯ One cup of skim milk or low-fat milk

- ❯ One to one and a half ounces of low-fat cheese or cottage cheese

- ❯ Eight ounces frozen yogurt (low-fat or fat-free)

Alternatives to cow's milk:

- ❯ Almond Milk – Low in calories, dairy free, high in calcium and Vitamin D.

- ❯ Soy Milk – Low in calories, high in protein and amino acids.

- ❯ Oat Milk – High in protein, carbohydrates, and fiber.

- ❯ Rice Milk – Least allergenic of all the non-dairy milks. Can spike high glucose levels. Low in protein. Not good for growing children.

- ❯ Cashew Milk – Low in protein content and calories.

- ❯ Macadamia Milk – Low calories, carbohydrates, and fat.

- ❯ Hemp Milk – Made from cannabis sativa. Low in calories. High in fiber and protein.

- ❯ Quinoa Milk – Gluten free. High in protein and carbohydrates. Low in calories.

- ❯ Coconut Milk – High in Vitamin C, folate, iron, magnesium, potassium, copper, manganese, and selenium.

⟩ Goat Milk – Has some lactose, so if you're lactose intolerant, you may not be able to tolerate it.

3.1f Fats and Oils

They say you should limit your fat to 30 percent of your calories. But who has time to count calories?! Know that some fats are better than others. Saturated fats raise your cholesterol levels and can increase your risk for strokes and heart disease. These are found in meats, dairy products, and some vegetables. Monounsaturated fats are healthier. They are found in olive oil, peanuts, coconut oil, and canola oils. Polyunsaturated fats are found in corn oil, soybeans, and sunflowers. Your goal is to eat low-fat foods and lean meats and fish.

Here are 10 high-fat foods that are healthy:

⟩ Avocados

⟩ Cheese

⟩ Dark Chocolate – high in fiber and antioxidants

⟩ Whole Eggs

⟩ Fatty fish – salmon, mackerel, trout, sardines, and herring

- Fish Oil – cod fish liver oil contains all omega-3 fatty acids

- Nuts – almonds, walnuts, macadamia

- Chia Seeds

- Extra Virgin Olive Oil

- Coconuts and Coconut Oil – Medium-chain triglyceride. Goes directly to the liver. Used for energy, increases the amount of calories burned, helps fight infection, reduces appetite, raises good cholesterol (HDL), moisturizes skin, and protects hair from sun damage

- Full-Fat Yogurt (look out for sugar content in some brands)

3.2 MANAGING CRAVINGS

Now you know what to eat. But you still want that cookie! How can you stop these cravings? Well, say no more. Here are a few tricks on how to curb cravings:

- Drink more water. Thirst is often confused with hunger or food cravings. Wait a few minutes, and the craving may pass.

❯ Eating more protein will reduce your appetite and keep you fuller longer. It can reduce your nighttime cravings by 50 percent.

❯ Chewing gum can reduce cravings and your appetite.

❯ Distance yourself from the craving. If you don't buy it, you can't eat it. Keep your house full of nutritious snacks. Keep a granola bar or nuts in your bag. Walk with an apple.

❯ If you plan your meals and snacks for the day, there is less room for deviation from the plan. You are less tempted to buy that candy bar because you have your cherries already packed.

❯ Try to eat every two to three hours in small portions. This prevents us from getting overly hungry, which is when we tend to snack the most.

❯ Reduce stress by increasing physical activity, meditating, and planning ahead can decrease your cravings. Stress releases cortisol, which can cause weight gain, especially around your belly.

- Get enough sleep. Sleep deprivation disrupts the normal flow of hormones and can lead to a poor appetite.

- Don't grocery shop hungry.

- When you do crave something sweet, substitute it with a fruit or dark chocolate that is at least 75 percent coca, which has antioxidants.

- Eat Greek yogurt, as it's high in protein and low in calories.

- Drink hot tea after meals to reduce cravings for dessert.

- Cottage cheese is high in protein and low in calories. It keeps you fuller longer.

- Lightly salted popcorn or vegetable chips can be substituted for potato chips.

- Trail mix and edamame are excellent snacks.

3.3 EATING ON THE GO

Many of us just don't have time to prepare our meals. We barely have time to grocery shop or we just don't cook. That's okay. We have to improvise. Have you ever tried a meal delivery service like Blue Apron, Hello Fresh, or Veestro? Some of the meals you may have to cook, others you can just heat up. Give it a try. If you're still hesitant and want to order out, see what healthy organic restaurants are in your neighborhood or look at the menu and create your own healthy meal. For example, I love Chinese food, but it is full of salt and oil. When ordering, have them put the sauce on the side. Get a main dish with vegetables and a side of brown rice. You can drizzle the sauce on your meat and vegetables. Voila! You just had a healthy meal on the go. If you like fast foods like McDonalds, order a salad with grilled chicken and a low-fat salad dressing that you sprinkle lightly on your salad. We don't have to go out of our norm to eat. We just have to consciously choose healthier options.

3.4 ALCOHOL

Currently, it is suggested that one or two glasses of wine or beer a day will not harm you. However, a recent global study on the effects of alcohol contradicts this statement. This study found that alcohol use was the seventh leading risk factor for premature death and disability among men and women between the ages of 15-49 globally in

2016.[6] It also suggested that there is no amount of liquor, wine, or beer that is safe for your overall health.

Until we all decide to quit, there are some healthier alcohols you can drink. (*Caution: This is not to promote alcohol use or to encourage excessive alcohol use. This is for those who indulge every once in a while.*)

The healthiest way to drink liquor is neat or on the rocks. Avoid mixers.

- Tequila – (one ounce) Agavins, the natural sugar found in tequila, is non-digestible and won't raise your blood sugar level. It can help lower cholesterol and help with weight loss. Gluten free.

- Red Wine – (five-ounce glass) Has compounds that have been proven to improve overall heart health. Also high in antioxidants.

- Light Rum – (one and a half ounces) Made from molasses, which can potentially reduce anxiety and help fight colds.

---

6   https://www.thelancet.com/journals/lancet/article/PIIS0140-6736(18)31310-2/fulltext

- ❯ Whiskey – (one and a half ounces) High in anti-oxidants. Helps to fight colds and inflammation.

- ❯ Gin – (one and a half ounces) Low in calories.

- ❯ Rosé – The polyphenols can prevent atherosclerosis. However it is higher in calories.

- ❯ Champagne – Lower in calories than a glass of white wine or beer. Has antioxidants that can improve your skin.

- ❯ Beers are high in calories, so light beers are a better option. Miller Light, Bud Light, and Coors Light may be your best options.

- ❯ Stout – (Guinness) Made from whole grains, which gives it its darker, caramel flavor. High in antioxidants, fiber and B vitamins. Low in calories.

- ❯ Vodka and Soda – (one and a half ounces) Sugar free. Low in calories. However, it has no nutritional value.

{ NOTES }

{ NOTES }

{ NOTES }

{ NOTES }

CHAPTER 4

EXERCISE

"Before you're old and weak, give it all you've got today."

—**Beres Hammond**

If you're like me, you make multiple excuses as to why you can't work out today. However, would you believe me if I told you that if you could fit a total of 30 minutes of exercise into your day, you could lose weight? No one said it had to all be in one sitting. You can break it up into shorter intervals, but it all depends on how intense your intervals are. The American College of Sports Medicine (ACSM) recommends that you get between 150 and 250 minutes of moderate to vigorous exercise each week to lose weight. You can break it up however you want. Making lifestyle changes is not about weight loss, it's about being healthy. Incorporating movement into your day helps build stamina, reduce stress, improve your health, and boost your immunity. If you lose some weight and tone up, that's an added bonus. You don't need a gym membership. You don't need equipment. As long as you have your body, let's get moving. Have you heard the saying, "Use it before you lose it?" It is that simple!

Exercise to be fit, not skinny! The only person you have to challenge is yourself. The only person who reaps the benefits is you. When you slack off on your routine, it only hurts you. So from now on, we are prioritizing ourselves and putting in the work.

So, how much exercise do you really need? That question depends on you and your needs. I don't want you to focus on weight loss. Focus on being healthy. Weight loss will follow, especially if you adhere to your diet. Exercise is the icing on top of the cake that gets you to your goals a little faster.

What kind of exercise should you do? There are four categories of exercise: endurance, strength, balance, and flexibility.

- Endurance training is aerobic activities that increase your breathing and heart rate.

  - Examples would be a brisk walk, jogging, playing soccer (football), tennis, raking or mowing the lawn, and dancing.

◆ Strength training makes your muscles stronger.

> ▸ Simple things like climbing the stairs, cycling, walking up a hill, lifting weights, using a resistance band, or workouts designed to use your own body weight can improve your strength.

◆ Balance training can help prevent falls, especially in older adults or patients with strokes.

> ▸ This would include tai chi, standing on one foot at a time, walking backwards or sideways, or heel-to-toe walking.

◆ Flexibility training allows you to stay limber. You stretch your muscles so that you can have more freedom for movement in your daily activities.

> ▸ Examples include yoga, Pilates, and tai chi.

It is best if you incorporate some or all of these types of exercise into your routine to get the greatest results. No matter how old or young you are, if you're able to walk or wheelchair bound, if you're strong or disabled, we can all find some form of exercise that will fit into our lifestyle. You don't have to create time to exercise either. We can incorporate it into our daily life. For example:

- If you're going grocery shopping, instead of parking in the front of the store, park at the end of the parking lot.

- If you're at work and have to take something upstairs, instead of taking the elevator, take the stairs.

- If you're watching TV with the kids, do some squats, push-ups, and jumping jacks during the commercial breaks.

- If you have 30 minutes or an hour for lunch, take half the time to go for a walk.

- If you have five minutes in between clients, try to hold the plank position or a low squat for one minute. That gives you four minutes to wash your hands, dry the sweat, and be ready for your meeting.

- If you're sitting in traffic, try stretching your arms, rolling your shoulders, and breathing deep to decrease the tension.

There are unlimited ways to incorporate exercise into your daily routine. You just have to get creative. You don't have to wake up early or change your routine. Just do it.

For those of you who do work out more regularly, switch it up, have fun, and do something you have never done before. Here is a list of some classes you may want to try:

- Boxing

- CrossFit

- SoulCycle

- Soca Aerobics

- Pole Dancing

- Ballroom Dancing

- Salsa Dancing

- Hot Yoga (hydrate before class)

- SkyRobics (SkyZone or any place with trampolines)

- Twerkout

- Swimming

- African Dancing

- Run on the Beach

- Rock Climbing

- Tennis

- Tabata Training

- Cross Country Skiing

- Jump roping

- Rollerskating/Rollerblading

- Online workouts (ex. myFitnessBabe)

What workouts do you want to try? Don't be shy! Have fun!

{ NOTES }

{ NOTES }

{ NOTES }

{ NOTES }

CHAPTER 5

PREVENTATIVE HEALTH SCREENINGS

"An ounce of prevention is worth a pound of cure."

—Benjamin Franklin

Before you start your new journey, always consult with your physician. You may be thinking, "Why waste my time when I feel fine?" Well, many ailments that affect us as a Caribbean community are silent killers. You do not notice the ramifications until it is too late and irreversible. Routine screenings are a great way for a doctor to check for disorders that can potentially be harmful later in life. You want a baseline set of lab tests to ensure no underlying medical conditions are lurking around. Also, if you have ailments, you want to know if there are dietary or physical restrictions. Physicians are here to help you stay healthy. Don't only think about us when you're sick. Many conditions are preventable. You also want to follow up after you have started your journey. Doctors love success stories, and we use them to encourage and motivate other patients. We love to see you go from being borderline diabetic to non-diabetic or tell you that we are taking you off of your blood pressure medication because your healthy lifestyle has resolved your blood pressure.

5.1 WELL ADULT EXAM

Both male and female exams start with a conversation about your general health, past medical history, surgical history, allergies, family history, and social history. Then comes the physical exam. Your history and age will determine what lab tests and imaging your physician will order. There are certain exams specific to men and women that are part of the preventative screening. However, everyone over the age of 50 should get a colonoscopy. A colonoscopy is a screening test for colon cancer. They have been proven to reduce the incidence of colon cancer worldwide. However, in the Caribbean, colon cancer mortality is still very high. Don't let pride, fear, or uncertainty be the determining factors between life and death. Get screened.

During your physical, we will also discuss your social habits, such as smoking, alcohol use, drug use, and sexual history. It is important that you be honest with your doctor about your history. Tobacco is the leading cause of lung cancer, which is very prevalent in the Caribbean. The rate of sexually transmitted diseases (STIs) is also high in the Caribbean. Some diseases, such as gonorrhea and chlamydia, can be cured. However, others, such as herpes, HIV, and syphilis, stay with you forever. If these diseases are not treated early, they can cause long-term complications, such as infertility, emotional turmoil, and chronic abdominal pain.

5.1a Male

1. Prostate Exam

   Prostates cancer is a serious health problem in the Caribbean and has one of the highest incidences of mortality in the world. It is often symptomless until its too late. A simple blood test such as a Prostate Specific Antigen test (PSA) and a Digital Rectal Exam (DRE) are encouraged. Prostate cancer in people of African descent is usually more aggressive and results in death. If caught early, it is treatable and potentially curable. Men, please put your pride aside and get tested. The screening test takes a few seconds and can save your life. What's more important—your pride or your life?

2. Testicular Exam

For many men, finding out something is wrong with their manhood can be more terrifying than death itself. However, don't let fear or misinformation hold you back from getting evaluated. Testicular cancer often affects young men. It is rare, making up 1 percent of all malignancies in men. It is more prevalent in white men than black men. It usually presents as a painless lump or enlargement of a testicle. An ultrasound can be used to evaluate the swelling or lump, and once found, it can be treated.

5.b Female

1. Breast Exam

Breast cancer is the leading cause of cancer deaths among women in the Caribbean and of Caribbean descent. Breast self-exams and mammogram screenings are needed to prevent this.

Women with a family history of breast cancer should start to get screened 10 years prior to when their first-degree family member was initially diagnosed. Every other woman should start getting mammogram screenings at 40 years of age. If you feel a lump, pain in the breast, changes in the breast such as dimpling or rough texture, or bloody discharge from the nipple, seek medical attention immediately.

2. Cervical Cancer Screen/Prevention

Cervical cancer is the second leading cause of cancer deaths among women in the Caribbean. This is certainly a preventable disease through a screening test called a Pap smear and with the advent of HPV vaccination. HPV, or Human Papilloma Virus, has multiple strains, and there are certain strains that can be contracted through sexual intercourse that can cause cancer. The vaccine is effective when administered to boys and girls prior to their becoming sexually active.

5.2 MENTAL HEALTH

Mental illness has a negative stigma amongst the Caribbean community. Those with mental health conditions may not acknowledge it and may not seek the necessary medical attention. Others who suffer from mental illness are alienated, live in poverty, and are discriminated against due to misconceptions from society. Limited access to care often prevents people with mental illness from living a productive life. Lack of education and resources to support those with mental illness are challenges that face the Caribbean community. Speak to your doctor about your emotions, thoughts, isolation, and lack of energy. They will have the necessary resources to get you the help you need.

5.3 VISUAL HEALTH

Blurry vision, double vision, or things floating around in your eyes are all signs that your vision is at risk. Seeing an eye doctor and detecting medical conditions such as glaucoma, cataracts, retinal detachments, and diabetic retinopathy early on will help you preserve your vision. There is a saying that "the eyes are the window to the soul." They are also a window to your health. Your doctor can tell you a lot about your health through the eye evaluation.

According to the American Academy of Ophthalmology, here are the top 10 tips to save your vision:[7]

- ❯ Wear sunglasses that can protect you from UV-A and UV-B rays.

- ❯ Don't smoke. Smoking increases your risk for cataracts and age-related macular degeneration, which can lead to blindness.

- ❯ Eat right. A diet high in green leafy vegetables and carrots should be incorporated. People with diets high in Vitamins C and E, zinc, and omega-3 fatty acids DHA and EPA are less likely to develop age-related macular degeneration.

- ❯ Get a baseline eye exam at age 40 even if you have no signs or risk factors for eye disease.

- ❯ Wear proper eye protection to prevent eye injuries while playing sports or with home repairs or gardening.

- ❯ Know your family history. You have a higher risk of developing age-related eye diseases if your

---

7   https://www.aao.org/eye-health/tips-prevention/top-10-tips-to-save-your-vision-2

first-degree relatives have cataracts, glaucoma, macular degeneration, and diabetic retinopathy.

- If you have any visual changes, early intervention can successfully treat certain eye conditions. Don't wait for this to progress.

- Make sure the eye specialist you are seeing can treat your eye condition appropriately. Ophthalmologists are medical doctors who treat the full spectrum of eye conditions. Optometrists provide primary vision care.

- Opticians are technicians who design, verify, and fit eyeglasses and contact lenses. Each one has a different level of training.

- Follow the instructions for care and use of your contact lenses. Do not use saliva or water as a wetting solution, and do not use expired solution. Also, do not use disposable contact lenses beyond their wear.

- Beware of eye fatigue, which is when your eyes get tired after staring at a computer screen for too long. This can be a sign of dry eye. To decrease eye fatigue, you can follow the 20-20-20 rule: look up every 20 minutes at an object 20 feet away for 20 seconds.

5.4 FOOT CARE

Your feet are the foundation of your body, which means keeping your feet healthy can help keep you healthy. Most people take their feet for granted until they feel pain or problems such as blisters or calluses form. Tips for foot care hygiene include:

- ❯ Inspect your feet daily.

- ❯ Wash your feet daily, especially between the toes.

- ❯ Trim toenails. Don't dig in the corners.

- ❯ Change your socks frequently if you sweat throughout the day.

- ❯ Do not trim, shave, or use over-the-counter medications to dissolve calluses. See a foot specialist.

- ❯ Wear proper shoes with good arch support.

5.5 DENTAL CARE

Dental care is extremely important, as your mouth harbors a lot of bacteria. Many of the bacteria are necessary to kill the germs from different foods that we eat. However, poor dental hygiene can lead to cavities, infection of the gums, and tooth loss. Bacteria can also enter into the blood stream and affect our heart valves. If you have a joint replacement, bacteria can enter from your mouth and attack your joint. It is important to manage dental care for those patients with joint replacements, as bacteria can cause serious complications with that joint.

Here is how to keep your mouth and teeth healthy.

- Brush your teeth twice a day.

- Floss daily and in between meals.

- Limit sugary snacks and drinks.

- Don't smoke or chew tobacco.

- See your dentist regularly.

5.6 HEARING PROTECTION

Hearing is as important as seeing. It is one of the major senses, and when gone, it may never come back. It's important to try to avoid loud sounds as best as you can. Caribbean culture is marked by music and festivals, so your hearing capabilities are essential.

- Some things to keep in mind regarding hearing loss include:

- Wearing ear plugs when attending loud carnivals or parties or when working with loud equipment. It has been found that your ears need an average of 16 hours of quiet to recover from one loud night out.

- If you enjoy music with headphones or ear buds, the general rule is to listen with headphones at no more than 60 percent volume for no more than 60 minutes a day. It is preferred that you use over-the-ear headphones rather than earbuds.

- Don't use cotton swabs in your ears, as you can damage your eardrum or push wax further into your ear. Your ears can clean themselves.

- Non-steroidal anti-inflammatory drugs like Ibuprofen and Naproxen can contribute to hearing loss. Furosemide, a common fluid pill, can also contribute to hearing loss. If you notice sudden hearing loss, ask your physician if any of your medications could be the culprit.

- Keep your ears dry after swimming, as moisture can trigger ear infections.

- Exercise increases blood flow to the ears and can help the internal parts stay healthy.

- Stress can increase ringing in the ear, or tinnitus. Increased adrenaline over-stimulates the nerves, blood flow, and body heat, thus contributing to tinnitus symptoms.

- Get annual hearing screenings.

5.7 SEXUAL HEALTH

Let's talk about sex! Sex is a natural part of adulthood. However, as we get older, some of our parts don't function as well as they used to. To preserve an active and satisfying sex life, here are some tips:

- Eat healthy. Avoiding high-sodium food can reduce blood pressure. Erectile dysfunction can come from uncontrolled hypertension, cardiovascular disease, or uncontrolled diabetes. Erectile dysfunction affects one out of every two men over the age of 40.

- Avoid smoking. Smoking releases nitric oxide, which can cause decreased blood flow to the penis and clitoris. In women, it also reduces lubrication.

- Maintaining a healthy weight allows you to have stamina to enjoy those passionate moments.

Obesity increases your risk for high blood pressure, high cholesterol, and diabetes, which all contribute to poor sexual health.

⊘ Reduce your alcohol intake. Contrary to popular belief, high amounts of alcohol reduce your ability to climax and maintain arousal in both men and women.

⊘ Communication is key between partners. Let each other know what your preferences are. Don't do something to please your partner if it makes you uncomfortable.

⊘ Mental health is important. Depression, anxiety, post-traumatic stress disorder, stress, or any other mental illness may prohibit your performance. Seek medical attention and counseling to help you get past your inhibitions.

⊘ Protection! Protection! Protection! It is great to have sex in that moment, but the lifetime of mental, physical, and emotional trauma that comes with contracting a sexually transmitted infection or getting pregnant unintentionally is not worth it. If you're not in a committed relationship where you both have been tested, please use condoms!

5.8 IMMUNIZATIONS

Immunizations are designed to help boost our immune system to fight diseases that have taken many lives. Everyone has their own view on vaccinations, but the ones that are recommended have been tested and proven to reduce deleterious outcomes. At certain ages, certain vaccines are recommended. Discuss this with your healthcare provider about the benefits and risks associated with taking each vaccine.

5.9 DERMATOLOGIC (SKIN) EXAM

Our skin is the first barrier of protection from bacteria. It is the largest organ and can be easily damaged by the sun. Though many of us from the Caribbean have excess melanin, melanin is not enough to protect us from the damage the sun can do to our skin. Skin cancer can occur anywhere, but affects mostly those sun-exposed areas, such as our ears, nose, face, neck, arms, and upper back. It is important to have your physician examine your skin carefully, as changes can occur that may not be visible to you.

Moles that tend to change are the ones you need to monitor for melanoma. Here is a pneumonic to remember when monitoring moles on your body "ABCDE":

Asymmetry – If you draw a line through the middle of the mole, both sides do not match and are asymmetrical.

Border irregularities – The edges are not smooth.

Color – Benign moles are one color. Cancerous moles can have multiple colors.

Diameter – Cancerous moles can have a larger diameter than benign moles.

Evolving – If the mole changes in shape, size, color, elevation, or bleeding, it is concerning for cancer.

{ NOTES }

{ NOTES }

{ NOTES }

{ NOTES }

{ NOTES }

CHAPTER 6

MODERN MEDICINE

"The good physician treats the disease; the great physician treats the patient who has the disease."

—William Osler

In today's world of modern medicine, doctors are more accessible than ever. I am not ignoring the fact that some doctors may not have an opening for several weeks. However, when I speak about accessibility, I am speaking of the world of telemedicine and virtual care.

Telemedicine is a great tool for patients, as you can have on-demand access to a provider. There are various forms of telemedicine, including video conferences, texting, or phone conversations. This means you have no excuse not to see a physician. Telemedicine is great for simple concerns, such as an upper respiratory infection and urinary tract infections, or to review lab and imaging results. In a rural hospital setting where there are no specialists you can have a telemedicine specialist such as a tele-neurologist determine if you need specific interventions for your stroke or if it can be managed with just medication. A radiologist in Florida can look at X-rays of a patient in New York. There are endless opportunities for virtual healthcare to fill the gap where there is a lack of access.

There are limitations with this technology. For example, if there is a true emergency such as a heart attack or ruptured appendix, you need to be seen in person immediately and assessed and treated appropriately. Also, you need the proper infrastructure and technology. Most visits can be done through an app on your phone or through a website on your computer. However, you will need Internet capabilities.

For the busy professional, mom, or international traveler, telemedicine may be a great option for you to keep up with your health. We are all looking for easy ways to stay healthy without having to wait in an office for hours. If you're interested in learning more about telemedicine or looking for a provider who has a virtual practice, feel free to e-mail drkelenne@mycaribbeandoctor.com or schedule an appointment through www.drkelenne.com.

{ NOTES }

{ NOTES }

{ NOTES }

{ NOTES }

FITNESS APPS

Each app is different, so explore different ones to fit your needs.

- Aaptiv – In-ear personal trainer

- Playbook – Work out with your favorite trainer or athlete

- Sworkit – Personalized workouts in as little as five to fifteen minutes

- Keelo – Quick seven- to ten-minute workout

- 7Fit – Seven-minute workouts with high intensity training

- Lose it – Calorie counter

- MyPlate – Nutrition tracking

- Trifecta – Caters to diet and workouts of Cross-Fitters

❯ My Fitness Pal – All-around tracking of nutrition and fitness

❯ Nike+ Run Club – Best for outdoor cardio

❯ Strava – Best for outdoor cardio

❯ MapMyRun – Search a list of routes to run in your city

❯ Pocket Yoga – Use if you need some stretching or meditation while on the go

HOME REMEDIES

- Try drinking the juice of a prickly pear cactus fruit to prevent hangovers.

- Did you know that you can use papaya to tenderize meats, as it has an enzyme that breaks down muscle and connective tissue?

- Capsaicin cream, made from crushed hot chili peppers, is a natural way to heal muscle and joint pain.

- Rosemary tea can make your hair healthier.

- Cinnamon is used to regulate blood sugar levels, lower bad cholesterol, and help control indigestion.

- Noni juice is an energy booster can be used to help treat fatigue.

- Turmeric can be used topically to treat acne and make your skin look younger.

- Bushes such as fever bush (lemongrass or citronella), cerasee, and zebapique are used for common colds.

- Cerasee can also be used to help treat diabetes, hypertension, malaria, constipation, and worms. The tea can be used externally for sores, rashes, and skin ulcers. In a bath, it can help with arthritis, rheumatism, and gout.

- Honey and lime mixed together are great for sore throats. Some islands add onion to the mix.

- Ginger tea is good for upset stomachs.

- Aloe vera gel can be mixed with orange juice and used as a laxative. It can be applied to the skin to soothe sunburn and can help with dandruff.

- Warm castor oil on a cotton swab can be applied to joints to relieve arthritis and other aches and pains. Heating the oil and applying it to the scalp can reduce dandruff and moisturize your scalp.

- Bissy tea (kola nut) has been used to remove poison from the body, stop vomiting, and relieve upset stomach, nausea, menstrual cramps, headaches, gout, high cholesterol, and diabetes.

- Cloves can be used for toothaches and can help relieve a runny nose related to a cold. Applying the oil of the clove to the forehead and temples can relieve certain types of headaches, especially those from a cold. It can also enhance the sexual health of men when used externally. Chewing on a clove is a great breath mint. As a tea, it can relieve nausea.

- Breadfruit leaves help to fight inflammation and may help lower blood pressure.

- When roasted, the fruit of the calabash tree can be used to treat menstrual cramps and induce childbirth. The leaf can be used to treat colds, diarrhea, and headaches.

HEALTH BENEFITS OF COMMON CARIBBEAN DRINKS

Mauby (Mavi – Puerto Rico, Mabi – Haiti and Dominican Republic) – Helps with arthritis, reduces cholesterol, treats diarrhea and helps fight against diabetes. When combined with coconut water, it lowers blood pressure.

Coconut Water – Perfect beverage to restore hydration after exercising, as it replenishes electrolytes lost during your workout. It contains, carbohydrates, fiber, protein, Vitamin C, magnesium, manganese, potassium, sodium, and calcium. It can help lower blood sugar levels. Because it is a good source of magnesium, it may help increase insulin sensitivity. It also contains antioxidant properties to help protect your cells from damage. It may also help reduce kidney stone formation and help reduce hypertension and cholesterol, thus reducing cardiovascular disease. The coconut meat (jelly) also can help with weigh loss, as it is a high source of fiber and me-dium-chain fatty acids, which help burn energy in our bodies.

Sorrel (dried hibiscus flowers) – Can be used as a di-uretic (gets rid of excess fluid) and can help with weight loss, blood thinning, lowering cholesterol, and lowering blood pressure. It is also high in vitamins and minerals with powerful antioxidants. It can be high in calories as it is often made with a lot of sugar.

Ginger Beer – Mainly made from ginger root. It can help relieve nausea and can possibly relieve inflammation. Ginger contains multiple oils, but gingerol and shogaol are the two associated with the most health benefits.

Guava Juice – Guava is a super fruit and has many ben-efits. It's full of B-complex, Vitamins A and C, minerals, calcium, phosphorus, iron, magnesium, and potassium. The fruit can help with weight loss, as it is high in fi-ber and has no cholesterol, making it ideal for a snack. It lowers cholesterol and blood pressure. It has antioxidant properties that can help fight against prostate, breast, mouth, skin, lung, stomach, and colon cancers. It can also boost your immune system, as it's high in Vitamin C. It also improves digestion and can help treat food poi-soning and nausea. Other benefits include the promotion of healthy skin and improved eyesight. The leaves can be used to make a tea that lowers blood glucose. It can also soothe tooth aches, oral ulcers, and swollen gums.

THANK YOU

Thank you from the bottom of my heart for purchasing and reading this book! This is my first book, and never would I ever have thought that this would come true. However, with changes in life come changes in your desires, and this has been a turning point for me. I hope this book has provided you with some quick tips and suggestions that have inspired you to change your life. You could have changed your diet, decided to incorporate more physical activity, or even decided to see the doctor, whom you have been avoiding for years. I count each of those as wins in your life. We can't get to busy for ourselves. Life goes on without us, so we have to make the best of the time we have here. Your health is your wealth. Cherish it! Reading this book is the first step towards improving your life the Caribbean way. Please let me know your feedback.

LET'S STAY CONNECTED

WEBSITE:
www.DrKelenne.com

FACEBOOK:
www.Facebook.com/DrKelenne

TWITTER:
https://twitter.com/DrKelenne

LINKEDIN:
https://www.linkedin.com/in/drkelenne/

INSTAGRAM:
https://www.instagram.com/drkelenne/

PINTEREST:
https://www.pinterest.com/drkelenne/

GOOGLE+:
https://plus.google.com/b/104307213832941000012/

YOUTUBE:
https://www.youtube.com/channel/UCwaWEhEv7rLX-GGX3PebJRw?view_as=subscriber

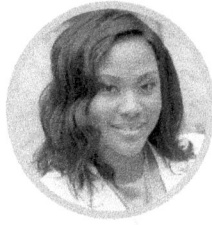

ABOUT THE AUTHOR

Dr. Kelenne Tuitt is a board-certified Family Medicine Physician, author, speaker, and concierge physician specializing in helping those of Caribbean descent. She was born in Trinidad, West Indies and raised in Brooklyn, New York. She helps busy professionals achieve optimal health on the go through her virtual platform, house calls, books, daily check-ins, programs, and services.

She has a world-class education with a bachelor's degree in Biological Sciences from Carnegie Mellon University and a Master of Biomedical Sciences and Doctor of Osteopathic Medicine from the Philadelphia College of Osteopathic Medicine. She completed her internship and Residency at Inspira Regional Medical Center in New Jersey. She has a passion for bringing the latest in technological advancements to rural communities both in America and internationally. Her philosophy is "prevention is better than cure!" In her free time, she enjoys traveling, dancing, and playing basketball with her son.

To connect, visit her website at www.DrKelenne.com.

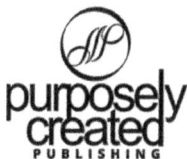

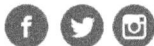